My Natural Birth Story

The Birthing Book I Wish I'd Read

ANGEL LEYA

ANGEL LEYA

DEDICATION

This book is dedicated to my children, for whom I labored to provide the best birth possible.

ANGEL LEYA

ANGEL LEYA

CONTENTS

ANGEL LEYA

ANGEL LEYA

ACKNOWLEDGMENTS

I would like to thank my husband for his amazing support. I wouldn't have been able to make my beautiful baby without him, and I wouldn't have been able to deal with the reality of raising a child without his help. He is the most beautiful, wonderful man a woman could ever hope for.

I would like to thank my mom and dad for their guidance in making me the woman I am today. I hope I can raise my beautiful baby (and anymore that may come in the future) as well as you have raised me. I want to thank my mom particularly for listening to me when I was sad or excited or being hard on myself. You have brought reason to my frenzied thinking.

I would like to thank my brother and his soon-to-be wife. You two have been so supportive and loving through it all. I am so glad the two of you are in my life.

Finally, I would like to thank God. Without Him I would not be able to experience this miracle called motherhood. He answered my prayers and gave me a beautiful, healthy, perfect little baby, and I am grateful that He trusted me enough to do so.

ANGEL LEYA

PROLOGUE

If you are pregnant for the first time, you're probably experiencing a myriad of emotions. Excited? Scared? Nervous? That was exactly how I felt. I was so unsure of how things would go. It was exciting to feel the baby within me, growing, kicking . . . but sooner or later it would have to come out. I made a decision early on that I wanted to go natural. The thought of a needle in my back was horrifying, but would I be able to handle the pain that came with natural childbirth?

I decided to write this book to get some things off my chest. What I experienced and what I learned gave me a passion to help any other woman who is pregnant, and especially those who want to birth their child naturally. I feel for all mothers-to-be; this is the most life-changing event you will ever experience. I hope my experiences will encourage you, make you laugh, and most of all, help you. The journey isn't easy, but you're not going through it alone.

Happy journey and Congratulations!

CHAPTER 1 - IN THE BEGINNING

I can remember the day I found out I was pregnant. My husband and I had been trying for about three years with no results. We had considered going to the doctor to see if there was a medical reason for our seeming infertility, but finances discouraged us from taking that route. Instead, we bought a book[1] on how to prepare your body to conceive and scoured the Internet for advice on how to improve sperm count and motility.

My husband and I had begun to suspect that I was pregnant around Christmas that year, but I was afraid to take a test. It seemed that every month the hope of pregnancy led me to take every little thing as a clue that I might actually be pregnant, so I would test, get a negative result that I reasoned could be wrong, only to start my period the next day. Then I would mope for a week or two until it was time to try again.

After three years of this, and nearly thirty-six tests, I didn't want to ruin Christmas by another negative test. So when it was about midway between Christmas and New Year, I was running late, and we decided it was time to test

---

[1] http://www.amazon.com/dp/0316024503/

once again.

I got up the next morning to do the test, ready for another disappointing result followed by another period. My husband wanted to be there for the results, so I started early, planning to wait the full five minutes before checking the results only to find that the test turned positive almost immediately.

I was stunned. I didn't expect the result to come so quickly. I ran out of the room to find my husband, and together we celebrated. The positive result was so much more important than being there to witness the result, so my hastiness was quickly forgiven, although he did keep bringing it up for about a week.

We called our family immediately, knowing that the soon to be grandmothers were particularly anxious for the day we would conceive. I was quickly cautioned not to get too excited about conceiving, since it was so early and the chance for a miscarriage with a first child was so great.

Still, I couldn't contain my excitement. We had conceived! Even if we miscarried, I knew that there would be sadness, but if we could conceive once, then we could conceive again. My fears of being barren were finally put to rest.

Although I can't prove it, I blame the pill for much of my problems conceiving. My husband blames a bad diet and mild dehydration for his end. Adjusting our diets, losing some weight, the addition of sperm friendly foods, and being able to let go of the desire for a child for a little while are what we contribute to our eventual ability to conceive, but that is a whole other story.

Once we found out we had conceived, the journey truly

began. Of course, we decided to take the precautionary route of keeping the pregnancy to our families and ourselves until we had hit the three-month mark. I remember thinking every day that I looked pregnant, that my little stomach was poking out more than normal and that someone might notice, but no one did.

This was odd in my opinion, since people had asked several times before, but now that I was pregnant, no one seemed to notice. Of course, after a few bitter replies, perhaps they finally got the hint: Don't ask me. I'll tell *you*.

In the beginning, you go to the doctor's office about once a month. This seems like an excruciatingly long time for a first time mother who wants to know if her baby is okay. The initial appointment consisted of a pap smear, collecting information, and determining how far along I was in the pregnancy. I didn't even ask whether they did a pregnancy test or not. They seemed certain I was pregnant, so I went with it.

At the end of the appointment, they had determined I was nearly two months along and the doctor said I would get to hear the heartbeat at the next appointment, since it would be about a month off. Of course, scheduling didn't really put me at the three-month mark, but I assumed I would be able to hear the heartbeat anyway.

Hearing the heartbeat for the first time was something I really looked forward to - audio confirmation of the life growing inside of me. I went to that next appointment, expectantly anticipating the sound that would change my life.

When the nurse put me in the room, her parting comment was that I wouldn't be able to hear the heartbeat until the next appointment. I was crestfallen, and as soon as she left, I started crying. Fortunately, the nurse read my expression and felt so bad that she got one of the other nurses to come in with her and try to find the heartbeat. They cautioned me not to get too hopeful – it was, after all, pretty early.

That precious heartbeat wasn't easy for them to find, as baby was still so low, but they did find it. I burst into tears yet again as relief and joy surged through me. It was true. I was pregnant, and now that I had heard the heartbeat, all bets were off. It was time to tell the rest of the world.

We did try to hold it in just a little longer, but someone finally figured it out. A gentleman from church noticed I was glowing. I never really noticed, although my husband encouraged me to put on extra makeup to try to hide the glow. We decided beforehand that if anyone asked, we would let the cat out of the bag, and so we did. It was official. We had a heartbeat, we had told people, and we were on our way to having a baby. Our joy couldn't be more complete.

CHAPTER 2 – OH, THE THINGS PEOPLE SAY AND DO

It's amazing the liberties people feel they have when you're pregnant. As my belly extended and it became more and more obvious, the strange comments and reactions ensued.

There was a girl in my workplace that was also pregnant, about three weeks or so ahead of me. I seemed to be gaining only in my stomach, while she gained all over. I would have been willing to gain in whatever manner necessary for this child, but she was a bit more self-conscious about her growing figure. I was shocked one day as she told me of a thoughtless but well-meaning gentleman who told her that she was gaining too much weight too fast and that she needed to cut back on her eating.

This enraged me, as the insensitivity and judgmental nature with which it was delivered was appalling. I'd been learning as much as I could about pregnancy, and one of the things I learned is that every pregnancy is different and as women's bodies vary, so does the way they gain weight. A taller woman may not show as much, while a shorter woman may look like she's carrying twins.

I told my friend not to listen to the man. She should

determine the health of her pregnancy by her diet rather than her weight gain, but I'm afraid the damage was done.

I got so many remarks as to how good and healthy I looked because I was gaining weight mainly in my stomach, but that really is no gauge of health. In fact, I found out early on that I wasn't eating enough. This will force the baby to leach the nutrition from me, which is not healthy for either of us. I was referred to the Doctor Brewer Pregnancy Diet[2] as a guide on what to eat each day. If followed, it will provide your child with the best nutritional support possible, which also helps prevent several complications.

Then there were the random strangers that would come up to me and rub my belly or comment on my pregnancy. Although I was happy to share my joy, being approached so casually by someone I had never met before was a bit strange.

There was one particular instance where a woman came into my workplace, spotted me, and sat down next to me, proceeding to excitedly ask me all about my pregnancy. I had never met her before in my life, and as she made her equally enthusiastic exit, I could only laugh, stunned by this random interaction.

Perhaps the cutest interaction was with that of a little girl. I wouldn't put her past around maybe five years of age. It was still early in the pregnancy and I was barely showing. She came over and lifted my shirt and began rubbing my belly. Although adorable, I did feel the need to cover myself back up again. Her mother scolded her for assuming I was pregnant, but I assured her that I was. That little girl must

---

[2] http://DrBrewerPregnancyDiet.com/

have had a sixth sense or something.

Inevitably, people would ask if I knew the gender, which you can't really find out until you are about 20 weeks along. Being our first child, it seemed to me that it would be more exciting to not know the gender of the child. I just wanted a baby, so knowing the gender didn't matter to me. Besides, I had heard so many stories of how the ultrasound was wrong and people had to return most of the stuff they had gotten at their showers.

I got mixed reactions when I would tell people I didn't want to know the gender. Some people said that was the way it used to be, and it was good. Many people said they didn't know how I could stand to do that or that it wasn't fair to everyone else not to know – like that should affect my decision. Still others warned that we would probably get to the ultrasound and change our minds. I know myself, and I was never one to peek at my presents, so I knew I could do this, and I did.

Then there were the comments when I would tell people I wanted a natural delivery. Oh, the moaning and wailing that ensued whenever I mentioned it! I got comments from 'I couldn't do that. I just want that baby cut out of me' to the ever popular 'Yeah, that's what I was going to do, too - until the labor started.'

First of all, you don't know me. I tend to have a high pain tolerance and am pretty good at pushing through rough situations when I know they're temporary. Besides, what do you suppose women did before doctors and epidurals were available? What do women in poor countries do now? If it were so terrible to deliver a child naturally, the human race would have died off a long time ago. At the very least, most people would have stopped conceiving after the first child.

No, wasn't fooling myself. I knew there was plenty of discomfort involved in childbirth. I knew it would get rough, but I had also learned that it doesn't have to be so bad as all that. At our first appointment, I mentioned that I wanted to try for a natural birth, and my doctor recommended that I seek the help of a doula.[3]

My husband and I were a bit skeptical at first. What in the world was a doula and why did we need one? We dismissed the notion at first, but when we found out her services were covered by our insurance, we decided to give it a try. The doctor assured us that the births that the doula had assisted with were some of the best, most beautiful births she had seen.

As my pregnancy progressed, the comments got more and more unbearable. Many times I would get the question about when I was due. The answer was quickly followed with a glance at my stomach and the comment, "Oh, I don't think you're going to make it." I carried big and all in the front, which made people doubt my ability to carry my baby to its due date. After hearing it every day from nearly everyone for a while, it got old. Every day I came in to work, people would act surprised that I had made it another day. They also seemed to think I was having twins. Eek!

Now there was a good chance that I was carrying a larger baby because of the diet I was on, but it seemed no matter how much I reassured everyone I was not carrying twins and that I would most likely make it to my due date,

---

[3] http://beachbabys.org/

no one listened. My mother carried large and got the same comments. The doctor let her go four weeks past her due date in the hopes she would induce naturally, which never happened. I was more concerned that I wouldn't go into labor, but if you hear something often enough, it can affect you.

The comments about my size started about a month before I was due, which meant I heard these comments a lot. I was proud when I made it to my due date, but I cried a little too. I was so disappointed that baby hadn't come by then, as everyone so eagerly had predicted. Of course, a due date is just an estimate, and with your first child, it's common to go a week late. It's also easy to get caught up in expectations.

Then there were the guesses about how big my baby would be. Now I know that a larger baby is not bad, and I expected to have a larger baby with the way I ate, but that doesn't mean I wanted others judging my baby or me. It was fun guessing at first, but when one woman started talking about eleven pounds, my tolerance kind of hit its limit. I knew the baby was not that big, and it was most likely a joke, but wow, was that rude.

There is a frame of mind that smaller is better to birth a baby, but I quickly learned that's not true. If your baby doesn't get big enough, your body won't release enough relaxing hormones, which means it is harder to birth because you won't widen enough to deliver. Also, if baby doesn't get big enough, your body may not get the signal it needs to begin labor. I also believe that proper weight helps the baby to turn when the time comes, although that isn't necessarily fail proof.

MY NATURAL BIRTH STORY

I also got the comment one time that having to birth a big baby could "wreck" my body. Now I know you can eat a lot of junk food and make your baby bigger, but I knew I was eating right for me and my baby. There was no reason to think baby would get bigger than it was supposed to.

I don't know about you, but in my opinion, major abdominal surgery (otherwise known as a cesarean) is more likely to "wreck" your body than birthing vaginally. The only exception is if your doctor does an episiotomy, which can cause major damage. I've had major abdominal surgery – a misdiagnosed and subsequently ruptured appendix – and it took at least a year before I felt I was one hundred percent again. I didn't want a repeat.

I got the comment "you must be miserable" through nearly my whole pregnancy, but I never knew how to respond. The thing was, I was never miserable. I'm not sure if the smile and glow didn't translate, or if people just wanted to believe that I was suffering, but this was a very frustrating comment. Don't assume that I'm miserable unless I tell you that I am. I got to carry through a hot southern summer, but I didn't spend a lot of time outdoors. I may have moved slowly, but it wasn't uncomfortable to do so. No matter what symptoms I had, I was happy to have them, since I was so excited to be pregnant.

Maybe I let too many cats out of the bag when it came to my symptoms, or perhaps I admitted to being tired too much, but the miserable comment came even from those I had never met before. Fortunately, there were one or two people who recognized my joy and encouraged me to continue in it. It was so refreshing talking to these people, and with their support, I could have happily remained pregnant forever – okay, maybe not forever.

Then there was the constant nagging about letting people know when we delivered. I know it was exciting. It was a mixed baby and everyone wanted to know the gender. I had every intention of letting everyone know when we delivered. I had a strategy – I was bringing my computer to the hospital, which had Internet. I would post to Facebook, send out emails and make calls. I even had a camera packed and cables so we could post pictures of the baby. Still, everyone insisted on calling me, starting about a week before my due date.

It seemed like we got calls every day. I was off the job by that point, so my mom and former coworkers were constantly being asked if I had had the baby yet. I honestly believe people thought we would keep the birth a secret from them. By then, it was tempting to leave everyone in the dark to drive them just as bonkers as they were driving me. In the end, though, I just couldn't do it.

While you're pregnant, you'll probably encounter your own set of annoying questions. Yet another reason the doula was so helpful. We had ten classes over twenty weeks in which I could talk to women who were excited to be pregnant, and I didn't have to worry about them judging, scolding, giving advice or making rude comments. We learned about the beauty of pregnancy and what to expect. It was such a nurturing environment, I could hardly wait to go to the next class. I could be completely exhausted by work that day, and even though I'm an extreme introvert, I would leave class feeling reenergized.

The best advice I ever got while pregnant? Assemble the crib in the nursery and ignore everyone's advice.

MY NATURAL BIRTH STORY

Your experience is not the same as someone else's. Your body will react differently to pregnancy, and you may have to deal with some things that others have not experienced. I never got morning sickness, but I got a pregnancy rash and pregnancy induced carpal tunnel syndrome. I got heartburn and congestion and some swelling in my hands and feet, but my stomach never formed a linea nigra.[4]

You and your baby are individuals with unique experiences. Don't let anyone tell you differently.

---

[4] http://bit.ly/1WYdjRE

CHAPTER 3 - THE DOULA

What is a doula? I can't speak for every doula out there, but ours was completely amazing. Pat Burrell is a beautiful African American who welcomed us with a hug and immediately began talking sense. As a mixed couple living in the south, we were grateful for her open spirit and lack of judgment. You would be surprised at how prevalent racist views, comments and attitudes are even today. She never saw our race, only two people wanting to welcome their child into the world in the most beautiful way possible.

The knowledge she's accumulated from years of experience was astounding. That's where I first heard about the Dr. Brewer Pregnancy Diet, which sold my husband on her services. He had been telling me for a while that he didn't think I was eating enough. She had facts and a chart and information that I could rely on.

When asked by others, the best way I could describe my doula was that she was a labor and delivery coach or coordinator, but she was so much more than that. She's so passionate about her services that she works as a nurse to support herself, since being a doula in this area was not yet paying the bills. She taught me everything I know, but she provided so much more than knowledge. She was a support, a counselor, a guide through this time of excitement and uncertainty. She helped me prepare for what was to come and to feel confident that I could accomplish my goals.

Her list of credentials was impressive, as she had been a nurse for about twenty years, particularly having experience with the neonatal intensive care unit, had worked with the March of Dimes committee, had experience with hypnobirthing, and was lobbying for increased awareness in her local community about the benefits of natural childbirth.

It's amazing all the knowledge she's acquired through her years of experience. She said it was akin to the way things used to be, back when a community of women would pass down the wisdom accumulated from all mothers before them to those who were to become new moms. Our society has lost that culture, as talk about sex and babies have become an embarrassing subject. Now people rely more and more on the wisdom of modern medicine, and the results haven't been so favorable.

Much of what I can tell you about my experience I learned from my doula, but that doesn't replace her. Knowledge can only take you so far, and there is no way I can impart to you the entirety of the wisdom she has accumulated. Beyond that, the emotional support and encouragement she and her associate Robin gave me during labor and delivery is simply irreplaceable. I would highly recommend the services of a doula for your pregnancy. I myself intend on utilizing her services for future pregnancies as well – it made that much of a difference!

I read a story once about a woman who had a terrible experience birthing her first child. She was induced because of high blood pressure then spent the night hallucinating because of a reaction to the pain killers the doctors used on her. The next day, exhausted and stalled in her labor, the nurse suggested that she go home, since her blood pressure had dropped. Instead, the doctor came in, saying he would only perform an exam, and instead broke her water. Her husband stood frozen, unsure what to do as she screamed for the doctor to stop.

Now this is not to say that your husband wouldn't advocate for you in a similar situation, but having someone experienced there who can remind, guide and advocate for you so that you can have the birth you want is irreplaceable. Again, I would highly recommend seeking a doula if this is your first child, as knowledge can reduce your fears, and fear will only make childbirth more painful.

CHAPTER 4 - DOCTORS, MEDWIVES AND MIDWIVES

As I determined how I wanted to birth my child, I had to figure out where and with whom my child would be delivered. Consulting the search engine pulled up very few options for my area. I knew someone who was a midwife, but she had moved, and was not an option.

Midwives are amazing, specializing in natural and home births. Their attitude is more laidback, encouraging the child to come as God intended rather than rushing things. Many times, they employ the use of a tub for a water birth, which I have heard is very helpful in managing labor pains. They encourage healthy eating habits as well as walking and bouncing on a ball to naturally induce labor. Their practices sounded like exactly what I wanted to experience in delivering my first child.

Unfortunately, midwives need the backing of a doctor in order to practice. This is to ensure that there's backup in case an emergency arises. While this is a good thing, if there is no doctor backing, as in my area, then you can't get a midwife to perform a home birth. I asked around a little, but my searching came up with only one possible answer, which made me a little nervous.

I decided to give up on the midwife/homebirth option, so I tried to see if there were any other options. An Internet search showed that we have no birthing centers in the area, so I had to choose from one of the three hospitals that were closest to us. When I ended up finding a midwife who worked at an ob-gyn office and delivered in a hospital, I was thrilled. I had found what I thought was the perfect solution.

As I learned more, I began to doubt if it really was the best decision. Part of what sold me on the idea of a midwife birthing at a hospital was that it just seemed safer. So many articles seemed to indicate that birthing at home, especially with a first child, was somehow more dangerous.

What I didn't realize was that there is a vast difference in the way you're treated, depending on who you choose. A midwife who births at home tends to have a more laidback attitude, a doctor seems to be more likely to come at you with scalpel in hand, and a medwife is somewhere in between.

I have to admit, I first heard the term medwife from my doula, who coined it. Basically, a medwife goes by the title of midwife, but has typical doctor training, more so than natural birthing experience.

Basically, I had hired a medwife. I believe the head doctor of the office provided pressure that influenced some of my medwife's actions, but there were certainly times when I considered looking for a different office. Being the kind of person I am, I didn't have the heart or the guts to move, but it all worked out in the end.

I've told you about midwives and medwives, but let me tell you why I absolutely did not want a traditional doctor to deliver my child. I can't speak for all doctors, of course, but I think many of them are motivated by money. Basically, the more you have done, the more money you or your insurance agency will have to shell out. For the hospital alone, a healthy vaginal birth costs only $3,000-$6,000 dollars while a cesarean costs $10,000-$40,000, depending on the area you live in and any complications that arise. In addition, with many of the practices that are in use today, complications are common.

Compare the United States with any other civilized country, and you will find we have the worst maternal mortality rates.[5] Not to mention that prematurity[6] is on the rise and it's the leading cause of death in newborns. With the rise in incidents of ADD, childhood obesity, and autism, it is a wonder that no one examines how infants are cared for when in the womb and the procedures employed to deliver and care for them. For all the advanced medicine and procedures we have, our doctors are not always doing us favors.

Let's look at what most women face when giving birth. It starts before you even get to the hospital. Gestational periods[7] can vary from 37 to 42 weeks (40 weeks is just the median and, therefore, the accepted period). Even with an ultrasound, the date of conception can be off by up to two weeks. Even with all of this information, as soon as you hit about 38 or 39 weeks, many doctors are on you to induce, telling you that waiting is unsafe.

---

[5] http://bit.ly/1HVa6va

[6] http://bit.ly/21ORiRy

[7] http://en.wikipedia.org/wiki/gestation

Thankfully, March of Dimes[8] has been able to increase awareness that women should wait for their baby to induce naturally, and doctors are no longer able to recommend induction before 39 weeks unless there is a medical need to do so.

If you do choose to get induced, there are a few things you should know. First, if you are not soft enough, they will have to give you a prostaglandin[9] treatment. Prostaglandin is naturally found in semen, so sex is a great way to ripen your cervix naturally. If your doctor needs to apply prostaglandin, however, you might be as appalled as I was to learn that they commonly use pig semen for this. Um . . . gross!

Then there's the Pitocin,[10] which is used to speed labor and delivery. Make sure you check that reference link out to get the full list of potential side effects and dangers.

Pitocin is basically a synthetic form of oxytocin. Oxytocin is a hormone released in response to love. This means kissing, hugging, massages and sex can all help get your labor started naturally.

In addition, the use of Pitocin can make your contractions, longer, harder and closer together, meaning you have less time to recover between contractions. There is also a greater risk for fetal distress, as blood flow slows during contractions.

Once they get you to the hospital, the doctor is on the clock. This means they need you to progress through labor

---

[8] www.marchofdimes.org

[9] http://bit.ly/1H7MCTr

[10] http://www.drugs.com/pro/pitocin.html

very quickly. They have little desire to stay with you as you labor, so instead they want to hook you up to machines.

A typical birth scene is a woman with an epidural, which means she can't move, and hooked up to a catheter and an IV, so they don't have to feed her or take her to the bathroom. They have two monitors on her at all times to check her contractions and the baby's heartbeat, further tying her to the bed. This ensures that they can sit and watch her vitals from a monitor at the nurse's station. If she failed her group B strep test, then she will also have an IV filled with antibiotics hooked up to her for the duration of her labor.

I don't know about you, but that is not how I wanted to deliver my child. The first thing wrong with that scene is lying down on your back. I don't know how many times I heard through the pregnancy not to lie flat on my back,[11] since it restricts blood flow. Why, then, is it so popular for delivery? This position is, I believe, the most difficult[12] to deliver from, since baby essentially has to come up to get over your tailbone. Trust me, pushing a seven or eight pound baby through the birth canal is not an easy task. In addition, lying on your back compresses your birth canal and slows your labor – exactly what you don't want to do.

I'm not particularly keen on the automation of a catheter and IV either. I've had a catheter once. I was out when they put it in, but I remember it coming out and that was not a pleasant experience.

Besides that, it's usually more comfortable to be able to

---

[11] http://bit.ly/1ihAxsQ
[12] http://bit.ly/1NCCKhb

walk and move around in the early stages of labor than it is to lie still in a bed. This meant an epidural was also out for me, which was fine, since I would rather deal with temporary pain than have a giant needle stuck in my spine. I seriously despise needles.

Given the option, I would rather be able to go to the bathroom on my own and eat solid food while I labor than be stuck in one position for hours.

My doula particularly recommended making a drink of orange juice, honey and crushed calcium to give you the energy for labor. It's also believed that calcium can help the muscles relax, reducing pain.

The antibiotics I find particularly disturbing. You're a healthy woman in a hospital, and you're being pumped with antibiotics. First, this kills your good bacteria and makes you more vulnerable to the abundance of germs present in a hospital.

I don't care what the doctors tell me, you can't say the baby – who is still dependant on my body for sustenance – would not be affected by the antibiotics. You've probably heard that antibiotics used on children[13] have been linked with antibiotic resistant germs, or superbugs. Recent studies have shown that there may even be a link between antibiotics and childhood obesity.[14]

If you plan on breastfeeding your child, there is a higher risk of developing thrush,[15] a yeast infection that can affect your breasts and baby's mouth and produces pain while

---

[13] http://abcn.ws/1LkS9B3

[14] http://yhoo.it/1HVbcXQ

[15] http://bit.ly/1S36pUv

breastfeeding. Breastfeeding is hard enough without the added pain of thrush.

In order to help speed along delivery, your doctor may employ different methods. Some of the ways they may attempt to do this is by breaking your water, attempting to widen your cervix with their fingers, or performing an episiotomy.[16]

Episiotomies are particularly frightening for most women. It's an incision made between the vagina and anus to help widen the opening for baby. This is only necessary if a vacuum or forceps are needed to help birth the baby. The unfortunate side effect is that it can easily lead to major lacerations, as it's easier for your body to tear through layers of skin as the baby comes out.

It's easier to heal if you tear naturally. If you want to try to avoid tearing altogether, it's recommended that you perform perineal massage[17] starting around week 36 of your pregnancy. You can also use perineal massages and hot compresses during delivery to further aid stretching.

If you want to avoid the typical hospital birth, then it's important to have a birth plan. This creates a written request for all to see, and shows the doctors and nurses that you're serious about what you want.

Understand that things do not always go the way you plan, but planning and preparing are the best way to help you achieve your goals. This is your pregnancy, and you should have the right to try it your way first.

---

[16] http://bit.ly/1WYalwq
[17] http://spke.co/1LkSm79

CHAPTER 5 - PREPARING FOR BABY

Since we spent so much time trying to conceive, it only made sense that I should do what I could to prepare for baby's arrival. When you think of preparations, I'm sure the first thought is getting the nursery ready, stocking up on diapers, and reading books about how to care for your newborn.

When I first found out I was pregnant, delivery was the last thing I wanted to think about. In fact, I was planning on putting that off . . . and then we met Pat, our doula.

From the beginning, she assured me that delivery did not have to be the horrific experience they always seem to show on television. You know the scene – the woman, covered in sweat, screaming for the epidural and lashing out at her husband or partner. Now I'm not saying there won't be some discomfort during labor and delivery, but it doesn't have to look like that.

There are so many aspects of preparation, and each one is important to the delivery process.

Probably the first she taught us was that of nutrition. When you don't get the nutrients that baby needs, baby will start stealing from your body. This isn't healthy for you or your baby. Not only does malnutrition[18] make you more susceptible to complications and premature labor, it can also have detrimental long-term effects, such as tooth decay. I've said it before, but it bears repeating. Check out the Dr. Brewer Pregnancy Diet, and make sure your baby's getting the nutrition it needs.

Of course, the next thing to talk about is exercise. You should consult with your doctor to make sure you're okay to exercise, but in most cases, you will get approval. Pat recommended that I walk about a mile a day for at least five days a week. You can work up to this. A good way to gauge if you're working too hard is whether or not you can hold a conversation while you're walking. If you can't talk, you're doing too much.

In addition, you should stretch[19] daily. Another way to prepare is by performing prenatal yoga[20]. If you seek an instructor, make sure they're certified to do prenatal yoga. By doing this, you'll ensure that your body is ready for the ultimate workout – labor and delivery! (Seriously, it's about the equivalent of running a marathon.)

You should get yourself an exercise ball. They can be used for labor, and sitting on it regularly will strengthen your core muscles, which will help with delivery. You can also rock back and forth on the ball to perform a pelvic tilt, which can help with back or pelvic discomfort. Rotating your hips in a circular motion while you are on the ball is another great motion, and it can help assist with the baby's

---

[18] http://bit.ly/1NCD3sg

[19] http://bit.ly/210St3q

[20] http://bit.ly/1MAAneU

progression through the birth canal during labor.

One aspect that may seem strange but is totally awesome is hypnotherapy. I'm not talking stage hypnosis where they convince you to quack like a duck. It's a deepening into yourself and relaxation. She gave us a CD with about an hour of script that went through the different chakras[21] of the body. This was to train us to relax, since stress is not good for the baby. We were instructed to listen to it every day, preferably when we were trying to go to sleep.

We were also given breathing techniques that can be used to help alleviate some of the discomfort of labor and delivery. (In four, hold one, out eight, or in four, out as long as possible.)

Massage is a great way to distract the brain during labor and delivery. Not the deep tissue massage that you would normally think of, but a soft grazing of the skin. The more often you get massaged, the better, and it doesn't feel too bad either! If you find your partner to be a little heavy-handed, you can have him use a feather to perform the massage. Massage has the added benefit of releasing oxytocin, a hormone that will help induce labor later in the pregnancy.

When you reach about 25 to 30 weeks, your doctor will probably have you do a one-hour glucose test. This consists of drinking a small cup of what tastes like a flat soda and testing your blood sugar level one hour later to see if your blood sugar levels are too high. The thing about this test is that they use a lower number than what is usually

---

[21] http://en.wikipedia.org/wiki/chakra

considered to be a normal blood glucose level.

My doctor told me I could eat like normal prior to the test and it wouldn't affect my blood sugar levels. I would encourage you that if your doctor encourages you to eat like normal, that you eat foods that won't spike your blood sugar levels, such as proteins and high fiber foods. A good breakfast would be eggs, oatmeal and an apple. Skip things that will spike your blood sugar level, like orange juice and whole wheat bread. Basically, if it's recommended for a diabetic, you should be safe eating it.

If you fail the glucose test, they will send you to do a three-hour test, which requires you to fast for twelve hours prior. This is not the best thing to do, in my opinion, since starving your baby for that long requires the baby to take from you, which, as I stated before, is not healthy for you or the baby.

In addition, if you're eating healthy foods, such as those recommended by the Dr. Brewer Pregnancy Diet, then your blood sugar levels should remain stable. There is a whole segment of information on gestational diabetes[22] on the Dr. Brewer site that goes so far as to suggest that it is not a real condition. If you had diabetes prior to getting pregnant, you will want to manage it as recommended by your doctor, but if you don't have diabetes to begin with, good nutrition means you won't develop it.

At about 35 weeks, your doctor will want to perform a group B strep test or GBS. This is a painless process in which they will swab the opening of your vagina, and in some cases, your rectum to test for the presence of GBS. If

---

[22] http://drbrewerpregnancydiet.com/id33.html

you fail this test, you'll be hooked up to antibiotics during labor and delivery, and if your water breaks, they'll insist that you go directly to the hospital. The fear is that the baby can contract GBS during delivery. This is not common, but in an attempt to prevent anything bad from happening, doctors do require the treatment.

Again, I'm not a fan of antibiotics in the hospital, or while pregnant. Prevention is, of course, the best medicine, and there are things that you can do to help test negative. The article from the Contrarion Mom[23] was very helpful (in my opinion – go ahead, check out the link). It provided information as to what to do to help test negative. It also has a list of things that may make you more vulnerable to testing positive, such as taking antibiotics, or if you had problems with yeast infections.

At about 36 weeks, you will want to begin perineal massage.[24] Again, this will help stretch and soften your perineum – the opening to your vagina – to help prevent tearing when the baby comes out. Your partner usually performs this but you can do it yourself. Basically, you use olive oil and your fingers or thumb to rub the perineum. Check out the link for more detailed information.

By 36 weeks, you should present your doctor with your birth plan.[25] This will give them time to review your plan and discuss with you anything they may refuse to do or have concerns about. For instance, my birth plan included the use of a birthing ball, but due to the hospital lawyer, I wasn't

---

[23] http://bit.ly/1HXoGNi
[24] http://bit.ly/1Mlm9AA
[25] http://bit.ly/1MRlQzd

allowed to use one once I get to the hospital, which is something they brought up at my next appointment.

Once you reach about 38 weeks, you will want to have sex[26] often. Baby was conceived through a loving act, and performing this loving act will also assist in bringing him or her into the world.

This works in two ways. First, the prostaglandin in the semen softens the cervix. Second, the sex itself, especially if you orgasm, can release oxytocin. Besides, once baby comes out, it will be at least six weeks before you'll be able to make sweet love to your partner, so try to enjoy the experience while you can. (And if you're unlucky enough to have severe vaginal drying, sex can be painful even after you've healed.) As my doula said, if a woman pregnant with twins can do it, then you should be able to as well. (The included link shows you some of the most comfortable positions for a pregnant woman to get it on. *wink*)

---

[26] http://abt.cm/1SX7DkV

CHAPTER 6 - THE CONCLUSION

I wondered what labor and delivery would be like. You see everything on television and hear stories from other women who have gone through it, and you expect labor to be excruciating. You expect to suffer, to need the relief of pain medication so bad that you throw away all your convictions. I personally expected to be mean and angry, especially to my husband. To be honest, labor was nothing like I expected.

I could tell labor had started at around 8 p.m. on September 1st. I was fairly certain I wouldn't have the baby that day, but the contractions were getting harder and stronger. I called my doula to let her know what was going on, and she said to call her if I needed her. I told her that I had a feeling that I would be able to get some sleep, and I did.

I went to bed around midnight that night as usual. I woke up once or twice to go to the bathroom and was fine, but by 5:30 a.m. the contractions were so strong that I could no longer sleep. I got up and walked around, ate and waited for a more decent hour before disturbing anyone.

My husband woke up around 6 a.m. as usual, and I told him that I thought the contractions were starting. We started timing to see the frequency, and found the contractions were about five to six minutes apart. I called my doula around 7 a.m. to inform her of what was going on, and she said she was on her way. I hadn't entered active labor yet, but we were getting close. She said to keep moving, breathing and to remember what she had taught me.

Finally, around 8 a.m., the doula arrived. We walked around, watched TV, ate some food, and waited for the contractions to get stronger and closer. I was able to maintain some level of comfort by breathing, moving around and shaking off each contraction once it was over.

At about noon, the contractions were coming close enough and hard enough that she felt it was time to go to the hospital. I was getting pretty emotional by then, as the flood of hormones released by labor took over.

Sitting in a car for the 15 minutes it took to get to the hospital was highly uncomfortable, but I was confident that once I got to the hospital I would able to walk around again. That was in my birth plan, after all.

Unfortunately, the hospital was not a safe zone for me. They insisted on registering me first, even though I was in a fair amount of discomfort by that point. I wanted to slap the lady who was trying to register us. It felt like no one cared that I was uncomfortable.

They rolled me in a wheelchair up to labor and delivery where they got me into a gown, strapped me to some monitors, stuck a needle in my arm "just in case," and proceeded to repeat most of the questions I answered at registration. They also checked to see how far along I was and found I was already at eight centimeters.

When I found out how far I had dilated, I was hopeful

that the baby would be coming soon. My doctor was unable to make it to the hospital for delivery, because it was Labor Day weekend and everyone in that office was on vacation. I had my birth plan with me, and gave copies of it to the nurses and the doctor that was on call, but even though my doctor had approved it, there were several things that this nurse and doctor were unwilling to do.

They refused to let me get up and walk, insisting that I remain lying in bed with the monitors strapped to me. This was perhaps the most devastating deviation from my birth plan. I had arrived at the hospital at about 1 p.m., but I was unable to deliver my baby until 8 p.m. that evening. Remember, lying down compresses the birth canal, which can slow labor considerably, and boy did it ever.

The nurses sat comfortably aloof, watching my vitals from their station, far from where I was. I was in the room with my husband and my doula and we were doing all the work for the six and a half hours that it took to get to the pushing phase. The nurse came in briefly to check my progress several times, and towards the end, the doctor came in to break my water. I'd been trickling, but my water had not broken yet. I believe that may have been due to the fact that I was unable to walk around.

Finally, it came time to push. I was surprised to find that I had no urge to push at all. I had heard so many stories about women not being able to stop even when the doctors told them to that I expected to feel the urge. Instead, it was just to the point that I could push, and pushing helped relieve some of the discomfort.

By then I was completely exhausted. I had been up since 5:30 that morning, and felt like I'd been going all day long –

which I had been.

I'd done my Kegels in anticipation of this moment, but none of that seemed to translate. All of a sudden, nurses and doctors surrounded me, and they, along with my husband and doula, were trying to instruct me on how to push. Commands such as, "don't push with your face," "don't push with your legs," and "push through your butt" bombarded me. The array of instructions was hard to sort through as I endeavored to push my baby out.

At this point, I just wanted the baby to be out of me. I wanted to meet my child, find out the gender, and to finally be done with the discomfort. I kept pushing, trying to do what I was told, trying to get the baby out. Finally, at the peak of my discomfort it was almost over. The head crowned, and within a couple more pushes, the baby was finally delivered.

IT WAS A BOY!

CHAPTER 7 - THE AFTERMATH

That first hour after delivery was magical. My perineum had torn, but with the help of a local anesthetic, I barely felt them stitching me up. I was able to deliver the placenta naturally and painlessly as my son breast-fed for the first time. I could have stayed in that moment forever.

My husband stepped out to make some calls, informing the family that we had a boy. This information had been so long awaited that we didn't want to make them wait any longer. As he made calls, I drank in the sight of my son. He was perfect, just as any baby should be. He was healthy and alert. I was so grateful that I had the support and strength to have him naturally. I knew I had given him the best start possible.

Because I didn't have an epidural, I was able to walk to my new room. It seemed kind of sad to me that this was such an unusual sight for the nurses. They marveled that I was up and walking, and that I had gone through labor and delivery without pain medication. How *did* women do this before modern medicine, right?

Perhaps what was hardest about having a baby, though, was breast-feeding. If you have access to a lactation consultant, I encourage you to use them. My doula is also a lactation consultant, and I don't know how I would've made it through without her.

It's normal when breast-feeding for the baby to lose some weight within the first week – up to a pound! Jaundice is also very common. When talking to a pediatrician though, they make it sound like this is the worst thing in the world.

The best thing you can do is to feed, feed, feed! As long as the baby is getting enough milk, you should be fine. The jaundice comes out through the poop, which looks green with black "seeds." If you just keep feeding, it will come out, as well as the meconium if that hasn't already come out.

Another fair warning: If you're fair-skinned, you're more likely to become tender or sore when breast-feeding. Fortunately, you can help toughen up your nipples beforehand with a simple daily routine. Take a clean, wet washcloth and rub back and forth across your nipple, then use a nipple cream such as lanolin to soothe the ensuing soreness.

My breasts were quite tender while I was pregnant, so I skipped this advice. I foolishly assumed that I would have no problems breast-feeding, since my mother didn't have any problems. Don't make my mistake, especially if you are fair-skinned.

Let me also warn you that it may take a while for you to get the hang of breast-feeding. It took me about eight weeks, although occasional problems kept cropping up. First, he wouldn't wake up to eat, so he wasn't eating enough, losing weight and getting dehydrated. Then he wasn't latching properly. It was difficult for me to understand the mechanics of how to hold him, even when using pillows for support. It seemed to work better when other people were helping me than when I was doing at all by myself.

What made it even more frustrating was that it seems like the formula option came up every time I complained. I wasn't willing to give up. Breast milk is the best for the baby, so I was willing to work through the pain, but that didn't stop me from crying and whining. I got discouraged so many times, but I'm glad that I pushed through. My little boy thrived, gaining plenty of weight, and I know that he is healthy, happy and better protected from germs because of it.

Breast-feeding was so painful at one point, that my doula suggested using a nipple shield. She also said that I should wipe my nipples with water, air-dry, express some milk to wipe over the entire nipple and areola and then air-dry again. This assists with the healing process.

Another problem I ran into was the squirming, fussing, and pulling off. This always seemed to happen in the evenings, and he was always unhappy if I didn't put him back on. Of course, he was unhappy anyways. This was difficult to cope with, since it was easy for him to hurt my nipples, which he did. I had to remain vigilant and patient as I waited for this phase to pass. They say the peak of fussiness is at about six weeks, so hang in there. Teething provided a new set of challenges, but by then, they were much easier to overcome.

I'm happy to say that having a child has many challenges, but in the end, it's all worth it. I couldn't be happier with my little boy, who brings me so much joy. In fact, my husband and I have already had another one!

Our bouncing baby girl was also delivered naturally. I was better prepared mentally, though I didn't do as much physically. I also found a better hospital – one that was

MY NATURAL BIRTH STORY

Baby Friendly – a program aimed at encouraging women to try to deliver naturally and healthfully. I had back labor, which was truly unpleasant, but I was able to manage that pain considerably. Thankfully, she came much quicker than my son – especially helpful since labor started in the middle of the night.

The second time around was also easier with breastfeeding. I'd experienced all the pitfalls, and knew exactly what to do when I screwed up. Yay!

In everything, I try to enjoy every phase. They grow up so fast, so none of the challenges that you face will last long. My mom says the first year is the hardest due to the lake of communication. If you're struggling through that first year, you're not alone. I actually found the first year of my second more enjoyable than the first year of my first. Chalk it up to toddler tantrums, but dependent baby feeding and cooing were a little easier to deal with.

There's nothing in the world that can compare to having a child. It isn't easy, and there isn't much you can do to prepare yourself for actually caring for your own child. You will laugh, and you will cry. You will worry and wonder and dream. Don't take anything for granted, because this moment will pass before you know it. I hope you take the time to enjoy your journey, because you only get one chance to do so.

Don't Forget To Leave A Review!

Your opinion matters, which is why you should tell others. I've made it super easy for you, too. Just use the link below to go right to the review page.

http://amzn.to/1O5ZSsW

It doesn't matter how much or how little you write, or even if you liked the book. I want to hear what you think, and so does the world. Reviews are one of the biggest factors that helps others decide if they want to read a book or not. Here's a QR code you can scan:

Now doesn't that feel better?

Sign Up For More

If you would like to know more about what Angel Leya is doing and when her next book is coming out, then go to:

http://www.angeleya.com/newsletter/

By signing up for the newsletter, you'll get updates on what's going on with the site and even the occasional fun email or freebie. You can opt out at any time and your email address will never be sold or distributed. Email frequency is about once a month, so you won't be getting slammed with emails (at least not from me). So what are you waiting for?

About the Author

Who is Angel Leya? She's a quirky girl who enjoys strange facts and putting love and magical fantastical things in all her fiction. On the serious side of things, she loves helping others, which is why she wrote *My Natural Birth Story*.

As you might have guessed, Leya is also a wife and mother of two beautiful children. (That's right, she went natural twice.) She's a transplant from rural New York, currently living in sunny South Carolina. Feel free to drop her a line anytime!

More information about Angel Leya and how you can interact with her can be found at:

www.AngeLeya.com

Also by Angel Leya . . .

Can saving a human really destroy her people?

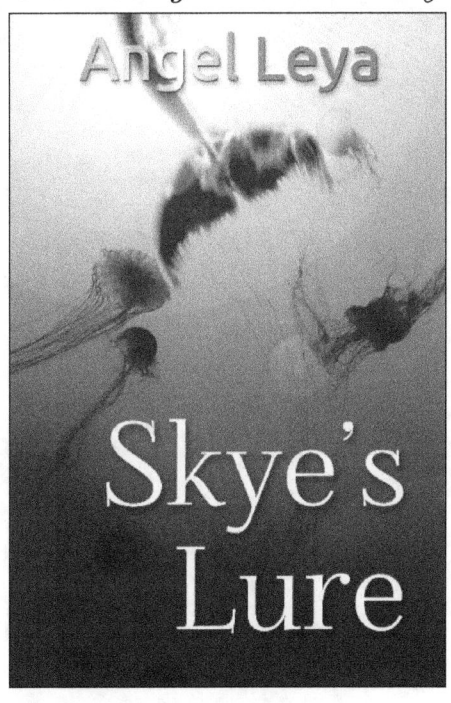

Skye is a good little Mer, following her elder's instruction and staying away from humans. But when a party ship cruises through her part of the sea, Skye ends up saving a man from drowning. When the ship comes back, so does she. Lured by the promise of seeing land, Skye boards the ship, but finds that her human friend may not be as trustworthy as she first thought.

Paperback $7.99
eBook $2.99

http://amzn.to/1XbyPNq

www.ingramcontent.com/pod-product-compliance
Lightning Source LLC
Chambersburg PA
CBHW062025280526
45787CB00005B/2214